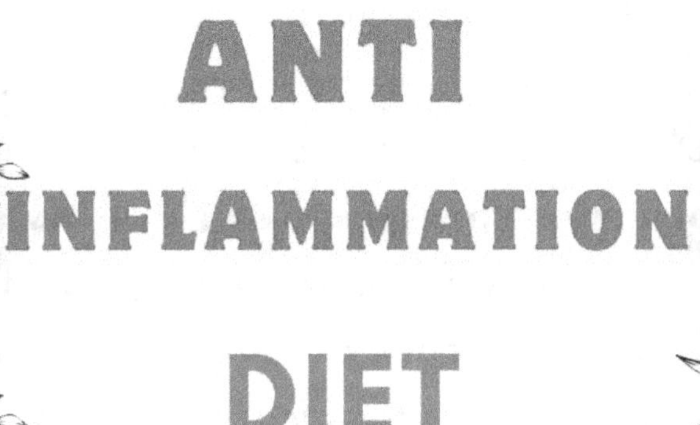

ANTI INFLAMMATION DIET

Cookbook

Eat Well And Feel Better With Delicious And Easy Recipes

Nadine Pierce

TABLE OF CONTENTS

INTRODUCTION

UNDERSTANDING INFLAMMATION

Inflammation is your body's natural defense mechanism against dangerous intruders such as viruses and bacteria. It functions similarly to your body's defense system, trying to repair injuries and illnesses. When you cut your finger or develop a bruise, you may have experienced inflammation in the form of redness, swelling, and discomfort. This is how your body repairs and protects itself. However, there is another sort of inflammation that isn't so beneficial:

Chronic inflammation. This type of inflammation can last for months or even years, and it is frequently undetected, with no apparent symptoms such as a swollen ankle. Instead, it simmers inside your body, slowly creating harm.

Why is persistent inflammation a cause for concern? It has been connected to a variety of health issues, including heart disease, diabetes, arthritis, and even some forms of cancer.

It can cause pain and discomfort, lower your energy levels, and make you feel ill.

The good news is that you can take action! Your diet has a significant impact on whether inflammation is promoted or reduced.

An anti-inflammatory diet emphasizes items that assist to cool the fires of chronic inflammation. It's similar to providing your body the tools it needs to mend itself.

We'll lead you through the fundamentals of an anti-inflammatory diet and give you with a treasure mine of tasty and simple recipes in this book. You'll learn that eating to minimize inflammation doesn't have to mean giving up flavor or enjoyment. It's the exact opposite. Our meals are full of taste and nutrients, making your road to improved health interesting and rewarding.

So, whether you want to avoid illnesses, lose weight, or just feel better every day, this book is your go-to resource. We'll explain the science of inflammation in simple words, introduce you to anti-inflammatory components, and take you through the process of designing meals that will make your taste buds sing.

THE FUNDAMENTALS OF AN ANTI-INFLAMMATORY DIET

An anti-inflammatory diet is not a difficult set of guidelines. It is, instead, a philosophy of eating that concentrates on certain foods and nutrients that have been shown to lower chronic inflammation in the body. This diet promotes the consumption of foods that have the ability to soothe the internal flames of inflammation. It's similar to providing your body the tools it needs to repair and defend itself.

DIET FOR PREVENTING INFLAMMATION

The following **fruits and vegetables** should be included in our diet: These are high in vitamins, minerals, and antioxidants, all of which assist to reduce inflammation. **Good fats** such as those found in olive oil, avocados, and fatty seafood, can help to decrease inflammation.

1. **WHOLE GRAINS**: Whole grains, such as brown rice and wholegrain bread, are high in fiber and minerals that improve overall health.

2. **LEAN PROTEINS**: Poultry, legumes, and tofu are good sources of protein that don't cause inflammation.

3. **SPICES AND HERBS**: Anti-inflammatory ingredients such as turmeric, ginger, and garlic provide flavor to your food.

4. **HEALTHY FATS**: Almonds, walnuts, and flax seeds are high in healthful fats and anti-inflammatory components.

5. **HERBAL TEAS**: such as green tea and chamomile tea, can be both calming and anti-inflammatory.

FOODS TO AVOID

An anti-inflammatory diet restricts or eliminates:

1. **PROCESSED FOODS**: These are frequently heavy in harmful fats, carbohydrates, and inflammation-promoting chemicals.

2. **SWEET DRINKS**: such as soda and sweet juices, can cause inflammation.

3. **EXCESSIVE RED MEAT**: While lean meats are OK, consuming excessive quantities of red meat may cause inflammation.

4. **TRANS FATS**: These dangerous fats can be found in a variety of packaged snacks and fast-food products.

White bread, sugary cereals, and pastries can all contribute to inflammation.

Understanding the fundamentals of what to include and avoid in your diet is the first step toward adopting an anti-inflammatory diet.

THE ADVANTAGES OF AN ANTI-INFLAMMATORY DIET

1. **REDUCED INFLAMMATION**: By eating anti-inflammatory foods, you can reduce chronic inflammation, which has been related to a variety of health issues.

2. **IMPROVED HEART HEALTH**: By encouraging healthy cholesterol levels and blood pressure, an anti-inflammatory diet can help minimize the risk of heart disease.

3. **WEIGHT MANAGEMENT**: This eating style promotes weight loss and maintenance, which is important for general health.

4. **IMPROVED JOINT HEALTH**: If you suffer from arthritis or joint pain, an anti-inflammatory diet will help you feel better.

5. **IMPROVED BRAIN FUNCTION**: Some research indicates that anti-inflammatory foods may benefit brain health and lower the risk of cognitive decline.

An anti-inflammatory diet, in a nutshell, is about feeling better and taking care of your long-term health. It's a straightforward yet effective approach to wellbeing, and we're here to help you navigate the tasty and nutritious path ahead.

KITCHEN INGREDIENTS

This involves stocking your pantry with necessary things, understanding what cooking equipment will make your life simpler, and mastering meal planning to stay on track with your anti-inflammatory quest.

1. **WHOLE GRAINS**: Stock up on brown rice, quinoa, and wholegrain pasta. They include a lot of fiber and minerals.

2. **CANNED LEGUMES**: Beans, lentils, and chickpeas are high in plant-based protein.

3. **HEALTHY OILS**: Choose olive oil and avocado oil, which are high in heart-healthy fats.

4. **HERBS AND SPICES**: Keep herbs like basil and thyme on hand, as well as spices like turmeric, ginger, and cinnamon. They enhance the taste and anti-inflammatory properties of your foods.

5. **CANNED TOMATOES**: These may be used to make sauces, soups, and stews.

6. **ALMONDS, WALNUTS, FLAXSEEDS, AND CHIA SEEDS:** are great for nibbling or adding crunch to your dishes.

7. **BROTH OR STOCK**: For delectable, health-conscious dishes, choose reduced sodium or no sodium added options.

8. **WHOLEGRAIN FLOUR:** may be used to make healthier versions of baked items.

9. **VINEGAR:** Balsamic and apple cider vinegar give your meals a tart edge.

10. **TAMARI OR LOW-SODIUM SOY SAUCE:** Excellent for adding umami taste to recipes.

ESSENTIAL KITCHEN APPLIANCES

- A cutting board and sharp knives
- Pots and pans
- Baking sheets and casserole dishes
- Blender or food processor
- Measuring cups and spoons
- Mixing bowls
- Kitchen utensils, Containers for left overs

CHAPTER 2

BREAKFAST RECIPES

These ten breakfast dishes provide a variety of flavors and ingredients to help you start your day on a healthy and pleasant note.

RECIPE 1

OMELETS WITH SPINACH AND TOMATO

INGREDIENTS

- 2 eggs are used in this recipe.
- 1/4 cup chopped fresh spinach
- 1/4 cup sliced cherry tomatoes
- Season with salt and pepper to taste.
- Cooking with olive oil

INSTRUCTIONS

1. Heat a little amount of olive oil in a non-stick pan over medium heat.
2. Whisk the eggs in a mixing dish and season with salt and pepper.

3. Pour the eggs into the pan, swirling them around to make an equal layer.

4. Top one half of the omelet with the chopped spinach and sliced cherry tomatoes.

5. Once the eggs are nearly set, fold the second half over the vegetables gently.

6. Cook for a further minute or two, or until the omelet is completely set.

7. Transfer to a dish, cut in half, and serve.

RECIPE 2

BANANA AND PEANUT BUTTER TOAST

INGREDIENTS

- 2 whole grain bread slices
- 2 tbsp of peanut butter
- 1 ripe banana, cut

INSTRUCTIONS

1. Toast the wholegrain bread pieces until they are golden brown.
2. Spread 1 tbsp peanut butter on each slice.
3. Pile on the banana slices.
4. To make a sandwich, press the slices together.
5. If preferred, cut in half and serve.

RECIPE 3

CHIA BLUEBERRY PUDDING

- Chia seeds (quarter cup)
- 1-quart almond milk
- 1/2 cup blueberries, fresh or frozen
- Optional: 1/2 teaspoon honey

INSTRUCTIONS

1. Combine the chia seeds and almond milk in a mixing basin. Stir well.
2. Stir in the blueberries and honey.
3. Combine everything.
4. Refrigerate the bowl for at least 4 hours or overnight.

5. Before serving, give it a good stir.

RECIPE 4

HASH OF SWEET POTATOES AND KALE

INGREDIENTS

- 1 peeled and chopped sweet potato
- 1 cup chopped kale
- 1/2 onion diced
- 2 garlic cloves minced
- 1 tablespoon olive oil
- Season with salt and pepper to taste.

INSTRUCTIONS

1. In a pan over medium heat, heat the olive oil.
2. Stir in the onion and garlic. Cook until fragrant.
3. Cook until the sweet potato is soft and slightly crunchy.
4. Add the chopped kale and heat until wilted.
5. Season with salt and pepper to taste.
6. Serve immediately.

RECIPE 5

YOGURT WITH BERRIES AND NUTS

- 1 cup strained Greek yogurt
- 1/2 cup berries (strawberries, blueberries, raspberries, etc.)
- 2 tbsp. chopped nuts (almonds, walnuts, etc.)
- 1 teaspoon (optional) honey

INSTRUCTIONS

1. Place the Greek yogurt in a mixing dish.
2. Garnish with the mixed berries and almonds.
3. If desired, drizzle with honey.
4. Plate and serve.

RECIPE 6

TOAST WITH AVOCADO AND SMOKED SALMON

- 2 pieces of whole grain bread
- 2 ounces smoked salmon
- 1 ripe avocado, mashed
- Cucumber slices (optional)

- Dill, fresh (optional)
- garnish: lemon wedges (Optional)

INSTRUCTIONS

1. Toast the wholegrain bread pieces until they are golden brown.
2. Evenly distribute the mashed avocado on each slice.
3. Pile on the smoked salmon.
4. If preferred, garnish with sliced cucumber, fresh dill, or a squeeze of lemon juice.
5. Serve either open-faced or as a sandwich.

RECIPE 7

HUMMUS AND VEGGIE WRAP

- 1 wholegrain wrap or tortilla (optional)
- hummus (two tablespoons)
- Cucumber, cut
- Bell peppers, sliced
- Carrots, cut into slices
- Spinach or lettuce, baby

INSTRUCTION

1. Place the whole grain wraps on a clean surface.
2. Spread hummus on top of the wrap.
3. Stir in the cucumber slices, bell peppers, carrots, and baby spinach or lettuce.
4. Roll the wrap up, folding the sides in as you go.
5. If preferred, cut in half and serve.

RECIPES 8

MIXED BERRIES AND ALMONDS SMOOTHIE

INGREDIENTS

- 1 cup mixed berries (strawberries, blueberries, raspberries, etc.)
- A half banana
- A quarter cup of Greek yogurt
- A quarter cup of almond milk
- 1 tbsp. almond butter
- 1 teaspoon (optional) honey

INSTRUCTIONS

1. Combine the mixed berries, banana, Greek yogurt, almond milk, almond butter, and honey (if using) in a blender.
2. Puree until smooth.
3. Pour into a glass and serve.

RECIPES 9

CUCUMBER AND AVOCADO SALAD

INGREDIENTS

- 1 cucumber, thinly sliced
- 1 ripe avocado,
- chopped Cherry tomatoes.
- halved red onion, thinly sliced
- fresh cilantro or parsley,
- olive oil, and
- lemon juice
- Season with salt
- pepper to taste.

INSTRUCTIONS

1. Combine the sliced cucumber, diced avocado, cherry tomatoes, red onion, and chopped cilantro or parsley in a mixing dish.
2. Drizzle with lemon juice and olive oil.
3. Season with salt and pepper to taste.
4. Toss the ingredients to coat.
5. Serve as a light salad.

RECIPE 10

TURMERIC AND ALMOND OATMEAL

- 1 rolled oat cup
- 1-quart almond milk
- 1 teaspoon turmeric powder
- Almonds, sliced
- (Optional) honey

INSTRUCTIONS

1. Combine the rolled oats and almond milk in a saucepan.
2. Stir in the turmeric powder.
3. Cook, stirring regularly, over medium heat until the oatmeal reaches the desired consistency.
4. Garnish with sliced almonds.
5. If preferred, add honey for sweetness.

Have fun on your culinary adventure!

Enjoy!

CHAPTER 3

LUNCH RECIPES

These 10 anti-inflammatory lunch dishes provide a variety of tasty and healthy choices to help you maintain your health and well-being.

RECIPE 1

QUINOA SALAD WITH CHICKPEAS AND VEGETABLES

INGREDIENTS

- 1 quinoa cup
- 1 can of drained and rinsed chickpeas
- Assorted vegetables (cucumber, bell pepper, cherry tomatoes, etc.)
- Dressing: olive oil, lemon juice, and herbs

INSTRUCTIONS

1. Wash the quinoa in cool water.
2. Cook the quinoa according to the package directions.
3. Dice the various vegetables.
4. Toss together the quinoa, chickpeas, and diced vegetables in a large mixing basin.
5. To create the dressing, mix together the olive oil, lemon juice, and herbs in a separate dish.
6. Pour the dressing over the salad and toss to coat.

RECIPE 2

CHICKPEAS WRAP WITH SPINACH

INGREDIENTS

- Wraps made from whole grains
- Fresh spinach leaves
- Chickpeas, cucumber slices, and red onions
- Hummus as a spread

INSTRUCTIONS

1. Spread a wholegrain wrap out on a clean surface.
2. Spread the wrap with hummus.
3. Arrange fresh spinach leaves, chickpeas, cucumber slices, and red onions on top.
4. Tuck in the sides of the wrap as you roll it up.

RECIPE 3

LENTIL SOUP

INGREDIENTS

- 1 cup green or brown lentils, dry
- Onions, carrots, and celery, chopped
- Broth de legumes à faible teneur en sodium
- Seasonings (such as cumin, turmeric, and paprika)

INSTRUCTIONS

1. Rinse the lentils in cool water.

2. Saute chopped onions, carrots, and celery in a saucepan until soft.

3. Stir in the lentils, broth, and spices.

4. Simmer until the lentils are tender and the soup is delicious.

RECIPE 4

SALMON AND QUINOA

INGREDIENTS

- Salmon filet, baked or grilled
- Cooked Quinoa
- Steam broccoli
- Avocado slices
- Dressing with lemon zest and olive oil

INSTRUCTIONS

1. Place the cooked quinoa in a mixing basin.

2. Arrange salmon, steaming broccoli, and sliced avocado over top.

3. Drizzle with a lemon zest and olive oil dressing.

RECIPE 5

BRUSCHETTA WITH TOMATOES AND BASIL

INGREDIENTS

- Whole grain baguette, sliced
- Fresh tomatoes and basil, chopped
- Garlic cloves, minced
- Extra virgin olive oil

INSTRUCTIONS

1. In a mixing bowl, combine chopped tomatoes, basil, minced garlic, and a sprinkle of olive oil.
2. Toast the pieces of baguette.
3. Spread the tomato and basil mixture on top of each slice.

RECIPE 6

WRAP WITH TURKEY AND AVOCADO

INGREDIENTS

- Wraps made from whole grains
- Sliced turkey breast
- Slices of avocado
- Lettuce and tomato slices
- Spread with Greek yogurt or hummus.

INSTRUCTIONS

1. Prepare a whole grain wrap.
2. Spread the wrap with Greek yogurt or hummus.
3. Arrange turkey, avocado, lettuce, and sliced tomatoes on a plate.
4. Tightly roll up the wrap.

RECIPE 7

SALAD WITH ROASTED VEGETABLES

INGREDIENTS

- Assorted vegetables (for example, bell peppers, zucchini, and red onion)
- Dressing: olive oil, balsamic vinegar, and herbs
- Mixed greens,

INSTRUCTIONS

1. Chop the vegetables and stir with olive oil.
2. Roast until tender in the oven.
3. Make a balsamic vinegar and herb dressing.
4. Toss the roasted vegetables with the mixed greens and sprinkle with the dressing.

RECIPE 8

TUNA SALAD

INGREDIENTS

- Drained canned tuna in water
- Greek yogurt or olive oil mayo with chopped celery,
- Red onion, and pickles
- Lemon juice with Dijon mustard

INSTRUCTIONS

1. Combine tuna, celery, red onion, and pickles in a mixing dish.
2. Combine Greek yogurt or olive oil mayo, Dijon mustard, and lemon juice in a mixing bowl.
3. Serve as a sandwich or with salad leaves.

STACKS OF EGGPLANT AND TOMATO

INGREDIENTS

- Tomatoes with eggplant slices
- Fresh basil, garlic, and olive oil
- Drizzle with balsamic reduction

INSTRUCTIONS

1. Rub eggplant slices with olive oil and garlic before roasting.
2. Arrange roasted eggplant and fresh tomato slices on a plate and top with basil leaves.
3. Finish with a drizzle of balsamic reduction.

RECIPE 10

SALAD WITH BLACK BEANS AND CORN

INGREDIENTS

- Drained and washed canned black beans
- Corn kernels (fresh or frozen)
- Bell peppers, red onion, and cilantro, chopped
- Dressing with lime juice and olive oil

INSTRUCTIONS

1. Combine black beans, corn, diced bell peppers, red onion, and cilantro in a mixing dish.
2. Toss with a lime juice and olive oil dressing.

Enjoy your tasty and healthy meals!

CHAPTER 4

DINNER RECIPES

These 10 anti-inflammatory dinner recipes have a variety of tastes and ingredients that will benefit your health.

RECIPE 1

SALMON BAKED WITH ASPARAGUS

INGREDIENTS

- 2 filets of salmon
- 1 asparagus bunch
- 2 tbsp of olive oil
- 1 sliced lemon
- Season with salt and pepper to taste.

PREPARATION METHOD

1. Preheat the oven to 400 degrees Fahrenheit (200 degrees Celsius).
2. Line a baking sheet with salmon filets and asparagus.

3. Drizzle with olive oil, then top with lemon slices and season with salt and pepper to taste.

4. Bake for 15-20 minutes, or until the salmon is well cooked.

RECIPE 2

STIR-FRY QUINOA AND VEGETABLES

INGREDIENTS

- 1 cup cooked quinoa Ingredients
- 2 cup mixed veggies (bell peppers, broccoli, carrots, etc.)
- 2 tbsp low sodium soy sauce (or tamari)
- 1 tablespoon extra-virgin olive oil
- 1/2 teaspoon minced ginger
- 1/2 teaspoon minced garlic

PREPARATION METHOD

1. Heat the olive oil in a skillet and add the minced ginger and garlic.

2. Stir Fry the mixed veggies until they are soft.

3. Stir in the cooked quinoa and the low sodium soy sauce or tamari. Combine thoroughly.

RECIPE 3

SKEWERS OF GRILLED CHICKEN AND VEGETABLES

INGREDIENTS

- 2 boneless, skinless chicken breasts (cut into bits)
- Vegetables (such as bell peppers, zucchini, and cherry tomatoes)
- 2 tbsp of olive oil
- 1 teaspoon dry herbs (oregano, thyme, etc.)
- Season with salt and pepper to taste.

PREPARATION METHOD

1. Preheat your grill to medium-high heat.
2. Spike the chicken and veggies.
3. Brush with olive oil and season with salt and pepper.
4. Grill the chicken for 15-20 minutes, turning occasionally, until done.

RECIPE 4

SOUP WITH LENTILS AND VEGETABLES

INGREDIENTS

- 1 cup cooked dry green or brown lentils
- 2 cups mixed veggies (carrots, celery, onions, etc.)
- 6 cup vegetable stock
- 1 teaspoon turmeric powder Season

PREPARATION METHOD

1. Rinse the lentils and set them in a large saucepan with the vegetable broth.
2. Stir in the mixed veggies and turmeric.
3. Continue to cook until the lentils and veggies are cooked.
4. Season with salt and pepper to taste.

RECIPE 5

CURRY WITH CHICKPEAS AND SPINACH

INGREDIENTS

- 1 can drained chickpeas
- 1 cup spinach, fresh
- 1 cup tomato dice
- 1/2 cup chopped onions
- 2 minced garlic cloves
- 1 tablespoon extra-virgin olive oil
- 1 teaspoon curry powder
- Season with salt and pepper to taste.

PREPARATION METHOD

1. In a pan, heat olive oil and sauté chopped onions and minced garlic.
2. Stir in the diced tomatoes and curry powder. Cook for a couple of minutes.
3. Add chickpeas and spinach and stir until spinach wilts.
4. Season with salt and pepper to taste.

RECIPE 6

STUFFED QUINOA BELL PEPPERS

INGREDIENTS

- 4 bell peppers, chopped
- 1 cup cooked quinoa
- 1/2 cup rinsed and drained black beans
- 1 pound corn kernels
- 1-pound chopped tomatoes
- 1/4 cup chopped onions
- Optional: 1/4 cup shredded cheese
- 1 tablespoon extra-virgin olive oil
- Season with salt and pepper to taste.

PREPARATION METHOD

1. Preheat the oven to 350 degrees Fahrenheit (175 degrees Celsius).

2. Remove the tops and seeds from the bell peppers.

3. Combine cooked quinoa, black beans, corn, diced tomatoes, chopped onions, and shredded cheese, if using, in a mixing dish.

4. Stuff the mixture inside the bell peppers.

5. Toss the stuffed peppers in a baking tray with olive oil and season with salt and pepper.

6. Bake for 2 hours and 30 minutes, or until the peppers are soft.

RECIPE 7

STIR-FRY TOFU AND BROCCOLI

Tofu and broccoli in a fragrant stir fry make for a quick and nutritious dinner.

INGREDIENTS

- 1 block of firm tofu, cut into cubes
- 2 cups florets broccoli
- 2 tbsp low sodium soy sauce (or tamari)
- 1 tablespoon extra-virgin olive oil
- 1/2 teaspoon minced ginger
- 1/2 teaspoon minced garlic

PREPARATION METHOD

1. In a frying pan, heat the olive oil and add the minced ginger and garlic.

2. Stir Fry the tofu and broccoli together until the tofu is browned and the broccoli is soft.

3. Cook for a few minutes more after adding low sodium soy sauce or tamari.

RECIPE 8

PESTO ZUCCHINI NOODLES

INGREDIENTS

- 2 medium spiralized zucchinis, spiralized into noodles
- 1/4 cup
- basil leaves, fresh
- a quarter cup pine nut
- Optional: 1/4 cup grated Parmesan cheese
- 1 tablespoon olive oil
- 2 garlic cloves
- Season with salt and pepper to taste.

PREPARATION METHOD

1. Combine fresh basil, pine nuts, grated Parmesan (if using), olive oil, garlic, salt, and pepper in a blender. Combine in a pesto sauce.
2. Cook zucchini noodles in a fry pan until soft.
3. Toss with pesto from scratch.

RECIPE 9

BAKED SWEET POTATO SALAD WITH CHICKPEAS

INGREDIENTS

- 2 medium sweet potatoes are used in this recipe.
- 1 can drained chickpeas
- 1/2 cup cucumber, diced
- 1/4 cup red onion, chopped
- 1/4 cup fresh cilantro, chopped
- 2 tbsp of olive oil
- 1 teaspoon of lemon juice
- Season with salt and pepper to taste.

PREPARATION METHOD

1. Preheat the oven to 400 degrees Fahrenheit (200 degrees Celsius).
2. Bake for 45-50 minutes, or until sweet potatoes are cooked.
3. Combine chickpeas, diced cucumber, red onion, and cilantro in a mixing dish.
4. Drizzle with lemon juice and olive oil.
5. Season with salt and pepper to taste.
6. Toss the chickpea salad with the roasted sweet potatoes and serve.

RECIPE 10

SOUP WITH TURKEY AND VEGETABLES

INGREDIENTS

- 1 pound of ground turkey
- 2 cup mixed veggies (carrots, celery, green beans, etc.)
- 6 cups chicken broth (low sodium)
- 1 teaspoon thyme dried
- Season with salt and pepper to taste.

PREPARATION METHOD

1. Brown the ground turkey in a large saucepan in a big pot.
2. Combine the mixed veggies, low sodium chicken broth, dried thyme, salt, and pepper in a mixing bowl.
3. Cook until the veggies are soft.

Enjoy your healthy dinner

CHAPTER 5

SNACK RECIPES

These 5 anti-inflammatory snack dishes have a range of flavors and textures to keep you satisfied in between meals.

RECIPE 1

GUACAMOLE WITH VEGETABLE STICKS

INGREDIENTS

- 2 ripe avocados are used in this recipe.
- a quarter cup chopped tomatoes
- 1/4 cup chopped onions
- 2 minced garlic cloves
- 1 teaspoon lime juice
- Vegetable sticks (carrots, bell peppers, cucumber, etc.)

PREPARATION METHOD

1. Mash ripe avocados in a bowl with chopped tomatoes, onions, minced garlic, and lime juice.
2. Serve with dipping vegetables (assorted veggie sticks).

RECIPE 2

PARFAIT WITH BERRIES AND GREEK YOGURT

INGREDIENTS

- 1 cup strained Greek yogurt
- 1/2 cup berries (strawberries, blueberries, raspberries, etc.)
- Optional: 1/4 cup granola

PREPARATION METHOD

1. Layer Greek yogurt and mixed berries in a glass.
2. If desired, top with granola.

WHOLEGRAIN CRACKERS AND HUMMUS

INGREDIENTS

- 1/2 cup hummus, chopped
- 1 wholegrain cracker serving

PREPARATION METHOD

1. Serve the hummus with wholegrain crackers for dipping.

DRIED FRUIT AND MIXED NUTS

INGREDIENTS

- 1/4 cup mixed nuts (such as almonds, walnuts, and cashews)
- 1/4 cup dried fruits (apricots, cranberries, figs, etc.)

PREPARATION METHOD

1. For a healthy snack, combine a range of nuts and dried fruits.

RECIPE 5

TZATZIKI WITH CUCUMBER SLICES

INGREDIENTS

- 1 cucumber, thinly sliced
- 1/2 cup Greek yogurt
- 1 minced garlic clove
- 1 tablespoon chopped fresh dill
- Season with salt and pepper to taste.

PREPARATION METHOD

1. Combine Greek yogurt, sliced cucumber, minced garlic, and chopped dill in a mixing dish.
2. Season with salt and pepper to taste.
3. Dip the cucumber slices in the tzatziki sauce.

Have fun with your healthy snacks!

CHAPTER 6

SMOOTHIE RECIPES

These recipes help you enjoy a nutritious and pleasant beverage that promotes your health.

RECIPE 1

SMOOTHIE WITH BLUEBERRIES AND KALE

INGREDIENTS

- 1 cup blueberries, fresh or frozen
- 1 cup kale leaves, trimmed
- one banana
- 1-quart almond milk
- 1 tbsp. honey (optional)

PREPARATION METHOD

1. In a blender, combine blueberries, kale, banana, and almond milk.
2. Puree until smooth.
3. If desired, add honey.

RECIPE 2

SMOOTHIE WITH MANGO AND TURMERIC

INGREDIENTS

- 1 cup mango chunks, fresh or frozen
- a half teaspoon turmeric
- 1 cup plain Greek yogurt
- a half-cup almond milk
- 1 teaspoon (optional) honey

PREPARATION METHOD

1. In a food processor, combine mango chunks, turmeric, Greek yogurt, and almond milk until smooth.
2. If desired, add honey.

RECIPE 3

PINEAPPLE AND SPINACH SMOOTHIE

INGREDIENTS

- 1 cup pineapple chunks, fresh or frozen
- 1 cup spinach leaves, fresh

- a half banana
- 1 liter coconut water
- 1 teaspoon chia seeds

PREPARATION METHOD

1. Puree pineapple chunks, spinach, banana, and coconut water in a food processor until smooth.
2. Stir in the chia seeds for a few seconds.

RECIPE 4

SMOOTHIE WITH RASPBERRIES AND ALMONDS

INGREDIENTS

- 1 cup raspberries, fresh or frozen
- 1 tablespoon plain Greek yogurt
- 1 tablespoon almond butter
- 1-quart almond milk
- 1 teaspoon (optional) honey

PREPARATION METHOD

1. Combine raspberries, Greek yogurt, almond butter, and almond milk in a blender until smooth.
2. If desired, add honey.

RECIPE 5

SMOOTHIE WITH PAPAYA AND GINGER

INGREDIENTS

- 1 cup of fresh papaya pieces
- 1/2 teaspoon minced fresh ginger
- a half-cup coconut milk
- half a cup orange juice
- 1 teaspoon (optional) honey

PREPARATION METHOD

1. Puree the papaya pieces, minced ginger, coconut milk, and orange juice in a food processor until smooth.
2. If desired, add honey.

Have Fun with Your Smoothies!

CHAPTER 7

DESSERT RECIPES

These recipes have a variety of flavors and textures that will please your sweet craving and benefit your health.

RECIPE 1

CHIA PUDDING WITH MIXED BERRIES

INGREDIENTS

- 1/4 cup mixed berries (blueberries, strawberries, raspberries, etc.)
- 2 tbsp of chia seeds
- a half-cup almond milk
- Optional: 1/2 teaspoon honey

PREPARATION METHOD

1. In a container, combine mixed berries, chia seeds, and almond milk.
2. Place in the refrigerator overnight.
3. If desired, drizzle with honey.

CINNAMON-BAKED APPLE

INGREDIENTS

- 2 cored and halved apples
- 1/2 teaspoon cinnamon powder
- 1 teaspoon (optional) honey

PREPARATION METHOD

1. Preheat the oven to 350 degrees Fahrenheit (175 degrees Celsius).
2. Line a baking sheet with apple halves.
3. Garnish with cinnamon powder.
4. If desired, drizzle with honey.
5. Bake the apples for 30 minutes, or until soft.

ALMOND AND DARK CHOCOLATE CLUSTERS

INGREDIENTS

- 1/2 cup dark chocolate chips (at least 70% cocoa)
- a quarter cup almond, 1 teaspoon of sea salt

PREPARATION METHOD

1. Melt dark chocolate chips in the microwave or over a double boiler on the stovetop.
2. Fold in the almonds and sea salt.
3. Place spoonful of the mixture on a tray lined with parchment paper.
4. Allow it to cool and solidify.

RECIPE 4

SORBET DE MANGO

INGREDIENTS

- 2 cups mango chunks, frozen
- 1 tablespoon coconut milk
- 1 teaspoon lime juice
- 1 teaspoon (optional) honey

PREPARATION METHOD

1. In a blender, combine the frozen mango chunks, coconut milk, and lime juice until smooth.
2. If desired, add honey.

RECIPE 5

BAKED PEARS WITH CINNAMON AND WALNUTS

INGREDIENTS

- 2 peeled, halved and cored ripe pears
- 1/2 teaspoon cinnamon powder
- 1/4 cup walnuts, chopped
- 1 teaspoon (optional) honey

PREPARATION METHOD

1. Preheat the oven to 375 degrees Fahrenheit (190 degrees Celsius).
2. Arrange the pears halves on a baking pan.
3. Garnish with cinnamon powder and chopped walnuts.
4. If desired, drizzle with honey.
5. Bake the pears for 20 minutes, or until they are soft.

Have fun with your delectable sweets

CHAPTER 8

7-DAY MEAL PLAN

These include meal plan for breakfast, lunch, dinner, snacks. Smoothie and dessert recipes. For 7 days.

DAY 1

BREAKFAST: Spinach and Tomato Omelets

LUNCH: Quinoa and Vegetable Stir-Fry for

DINNER: Baked Salmon with Asparagus

SNACK: Guacamole with Veggie Sticks

SMOOTHIE: Blueberries and kale Smoothie

DESSERT: Chia Pudding with Mixed Berries

DAY 2

BREAKFAST: Peanut Butter and Banana Toast

LUNCH: Curry with chickpeas and spinach for

DINNER: Soup with lentils and vegetables

SNACK: Berry and Greek Yogurt

SMOOTHIE: Mango and Turmeric Smoothie

DESSERT: Cinnamon-Baked Apple

DAY 3

BREAKFAST: Sweet Potato and Kale Hash

LUNCH: Grilled chicken and vegetable skewers

DINNER: Quinoa Stuffed Bell Peppers

SNACK: Hummus with wholegrain crackers as a

SMOOTHIE: Pineapple and Spinach Smoothie

DESSERT: Dark Chocolate and Almond Clusters

DAY 4

BREAKFAST: Blueberry and Kale Smoothie

LUNCH: Soup with lentils and vegetables for

DINNER: Stir-fried Tofu with Broccoli

SNACKS: Mixed Nuts and Dried Fruit

SMOOTHIE: Raspberry and Almond Smoothie

DESSERT: Mango Sorbet dessert

DAY 5

BREAKFAST: Greek Yogurt with Berries and Nuts

LUNCH: Quinoa and Vegetable Stir-Fry for

DINNER: Zucchini Noodles with Pesto

SNACK: Cucumber slices with Tzatziki

SMOOTHIE: papaya and ginger Smoothie

DESSERT: Baked Pears with Cinnamon and Walnuts

DAY 6

BREAKFAST: Avocado and Smoked Salmon Toast

LUNCH: Baked Sweet Potato with Chickpea Salad

DINNER: Soup with turkey and vegetables

SNACK: Dark Chocolate and Almond Clusters

SMOOTHIE: Mixed Berry Chia Pudding Smoothie

DESSERT: Dark Chocolate and Almond Clusters

DAY 7

BREAKFAST: Almond and Turmeric Oatmeal

LUNCH: Stir-fried Tofu and Broccoli

SNACK: Mixed Nuts and Dried Fruit

DINNER: Cucumber Slices with Tzatziki

SMOOTHIE: papaya and ginger Smoothie

DESSERT: Baked Pears with Cinnamon and Walnuts

Have fun on your path to a healthy living!

CONCLUSION

You've taken a fantastic journey in your pursuit of a better, inflammation-free lifestyle. You've equipped yourself with information, accepted the nourishing potential of anti-inflammatory foods, and gained a better understanding of how your dietary choices affect your overall health. This route is about recovering control of your health, increasing your energy, and assuring a brighter future.

Remember that every step you take along this path is a step toward a more vibrant, energetic, and robust self. Your dedication to an anti-inflammatory diet is more than just what you eat; it is a commitment to a life full of energy, fewer health issues, and the ability to cherish each moment to the fullest.

We'd love to hear about your wonderful trip. Your review and evaluations are vital not only to us, but also to others who are going on this transforming journey. Your experiences can inspire, guide, and create a supportive network for those who are pursuing similar health and wellness objectives.

If you have any concerns, need assistance, or simply want to share your successes and struggles, please contact our dedicated support staff at nadinepiercehelpdesk@gmail.com We are happy to help you in any manner we can.

Finally, we'd want to offer our deepest appreciation for joining us on our journey into the realm of anti-inflammatory diet. Your dedication to your health is admirable, and your decision to prioritize it is admirable.

Thank you for joining us on this adventure. Here's to a healthy, inflammation-free future!